Zuo Yuezi
An American Mother's Guide to Chinese Postpartum Recovery

Guang Ming Whitley

First Edition Copyright © 2012 Guang Ming Whitley
Second Edition Copyright © 2013 Guang Ming Whitley
Third Edition Copyright © 2016 Guang Ming Whitley

Illustrations: Kai Tsu Easlon
Cover Art: Erica Hardy
Cover Layout: Hsien Ming Easlon

All rights reserved.

ISBN-13: 978-1533081148
ISBN-10: 153308114X

DEDICATION

For my mother, who made all of this possible.

CONTENTS

	Introduction	1
1	The Basics	11
2	Lifestyle Commandments	14
3	Diet Commandments	32
4	Exercises	37
5	Food List and Recipes	68
	Recipe Index	102

Introduction

I wrote the first edition of my guide to *zuo yuezi* while hooked to a breast pump. To an exhausted mother of infant twins, a 21-month old boy, and a 3.5 year old girl, the pump's hypnotic whir was a dangerous thing. Hearing too many stories about spilled milk, I decided to stay awake by writing in 30-minute sessions. At midnight. And 3 AM. And 6 AM. And so on.

When I started doing *zuo yuezi* (pronounced like z-war yeah-dz if war and yeah were said by someone with a heavy Boston accent), I had many friends who were curious about it. They wanted to know if I got bored after 30 days staying home with no visitors (55 days for the twins). They wanted to know about boiling pig feet with rice-wine soaked black beans and exercises my immigrant mother titled, "Get Rid of Big

Fat Butt" and "Tighten Vergina Mustle." I had an email ready to go with the basics, and I sent it out to many a pregnant friend. Some of them wanted more. Detailed recipes. Better explanations of how to do the exercises and how to wear the cotton tummy wrap. I had a few problems with this.

    1. Chinese people don't use recipes.

    2. It's hard to explain some things without a visual, and there was no way I was going to film myself using both hands to rub my belly from navel to pubic bone.

    So while doing *zuo yuezi* with the twins, I asked my mother to describe all the exercises and make illustrations to go with them. I also observed her in the kitchen and took extensive notes, creating recipes to account for instructions like: add ginger until it tastes good. As I put the guide together, I deliberately made it succinct. Mamas don't have time to sift through the padding to find nuggets of actual information!

    Fast forward four years, and my guide has been used by American-born Chinese women, Caucasian women married to Chinese men, Chinese women who were adopted into non-Chinese families, women of varied backgrounds seeking a holistic way to recover from the trauma of childbirth, and more. Several doulas have told me they keep my book in their lending library, and a few new moms, who admitted they couldn't stomach all the recipes, said the guide served as a reminder that self-care is important.

Once my guide was published, I switched focus to other projects (like raising four children). Then I made a new friend over the shared experience of pushing our kids on swings at a local playground. Maria White Mebane is an award-winning short filmmaker, a ceramic artist, a survivor of postpartum depression, and a champion of women's postpartum mental health. Maria was so open about her own struggle that I felt comfortable sharing the real reason why I chose to engage in the ancient Chinese postpartum practice of *zuo yuezi*: My mother was hospitalized for postpartum psychosis a few months after I was born. Knowing this, I wanted to do everything in my power to reduce my chances of postpartum mental illness.

I did not share my mother's story in the first edition of this guide. She wasn't ready to tell it, and she didn't think it was important. Maria thought otherwise, encouraging me to ask my mother if she would let me tell her story. My mother bravely agreed. While her postpartum psychosis was never a secret in our home, I had only heard bits and pieces. To hear my parents talk about it openly, from start to finish, was heart-wrenching. I am so thankful she survived. I am so thankful I survived.

My mother emigrated from Taiwan to the

United States at the age of 26, moving to Texas, where her two older sisters lived. Her eldest sister had started a gift shop and her middle sister had opened a restaurant. At first, she lived with her middle sister's family. She worked in their restaurant and babysat her new niece when she wasn't working.

Several months later, her eldest sister sat her down and gave her a choice. My mother could stay in Texas, or she could move to California to live with her sister's mother-in-law, a Caucasian woman who had agreed to rent her a room and help her find an unskilled job. For despite my mother's college education and years teaching high school math in Taiwan, her broken English limited her opportunities in the United States. If she went, she would have an opportunity to build her own American dream. If she stayed, she would just help her sisters fulfill theirs.

As her eldest sister had been the one to sponsor her green card, and had been a de facto parent since the death of their father over twenty years before, my mother decided to go. When her sister's mother-in-law invited her to attend church, my mother recalled the missionaries of her youth, with their pale skin and gifts of colorful used Christmas cards. She had kept the Christmas cards in a shoebox under her bed for years. So she went to church and sat in a pew, dozing during every sermon because she couldn't understand half the words. A couple of months later, she met my dad at the church's singles beach party. He invited her over for lunch the next Sunday, and three weeks later they were engaged. Two months after that, they married. Almost forty years later, my parents are still married; though they always said I should never do something so foolish – they were just fortunate.

My parents have always been pretty content with one another. When they first married, in fact, they had almost no social circle. They went to church regularly, where my mother explored her developing faith. But they didn't really socialize with anyone outside of church activities. They could talk to each other for hours. They missed freeway exits and the start times of movies, and didn't care because they enjoyed each other's company so much.

On their one-year anniversary, they started trying for a family. Almost nine months to the day later, I was born. It was a difficult labor, the natural result of a five-foot-tall Chinese woman making a baby with a six-foot-tall Caucasian man. After 36 hours, the doctors delivered me by emergency C-section. The day after they sent us home, my father went right back to work. My mother was left alone with me, and her isolation became apparent. She had no car, no job, no family in the state, no friends other than my father, and a colicky baby. Then her grasp on reality began to fade.

While my mother tried to recover from an

arduous labor and a six-inch vertical wound in her abdomen, I cried any time I wasn't held. My dad tried to be supportive. Every evening after work he would take me, and we would nap together in a rocking chair. Then he would go to bed with a happy heart and sleep like the dead. Though I allegedly woke the neighbors with my crying, I could not rouse my father. He was wholly unaware that my mother was nervously in bed beside him, waiting for me to cry because she was convinced I would start the minute she fell asleep.

She slept maybe an hour or two each night and towards the end stopped sleeping entirely. She began seeing things in the linoleum floor, believing that she was flying in the air and the rectangular patterns in the tiles were buildings and roads beneath her. She heard indistinct voices and music in the house when the TV and radio were off. She believed that angels were appearing to her, giving her special messages. She had always loved art, and spent hours in the middle of the night doing Chinese brush paintings. She thought they were beautiful and complex. My father says they were like the drawings of a young child. She papered the walls of the house with them.

Perhaps it was the era, the newness of their relationship, or the lack of an outside observer to notice the change in my mother, but it took almost two months for my father to realize something was seriously wrong. He came home from work one day to find me alone in the house, screaming in my crib. It was unclear how long I had been there or how long I had been crying. My mother was outside, painting. She told him it was fine, the angels told her they were taking care of me.

That evening, my mother was diagnosed with postpartum psychosis and admitted to the hospital. With the help of medication, she slept for 72 hours straight. When she awoke, her hallucinations became sinister. She saw demons, aliens, and malformed creatures dancing at the foot of her bed. She tried to banish them in the name of God. My mother spent 10 days in the psychiatric ward before she was discharged, and returned home to help from her mother and mother-in-law.

Part of her recovery was breaking her isolation. While my mother was in the hospital, various church members came to visit. One visitor brought a Chinese woman with her, thinking it might be nice for my mom to speak to someone in her native language. That kind gesture changed my mother's life. The Chinese woman was an architect, and heavily involved in the nascent Chinese community of the San Gabriel Valley – a community my mother didn't know existed. The woman learned she was a teacher and helped my mother get a job at the local Chinese language school on Saturday mornings. She made friends. She learned about free Mommy & Me classes and library activities for children. She started taking art courses at a local adult school. She preserved her own identity as an artist and a teacher, even as she made her primary focus caring for me.

When my brother was born two years later, my parents took preventative measures. They were able to hire someone to assist my mother during the day and my father made sure she got enough sleep. With these changes, she did not suffer a second episode of postpartum psychosis.

To this day, my mother's approach to life is filled with so much joy. I am grateful to be her daughter, and grateful my children have such a strong and wonderful grandmother.

I don't remember when I first learned what happened after I was born. It seems like it was always there, a knowledge that my mother had been hospitalized. That I cried more than the average baby. That she'd had hallucinations. Even as a teenager, whenever I thought about getting married or having a child, I worried about my mother's postpartum psychosis. I knew there was a hereditary aspect and I was terrified that I would get it. I wondered if it was something I should tell my future husband, so he could look for signs. Or if it were something to hide from him, so he would still want to make babies with me. I wondered if there was anything I could do to stop it from happening.

I didn't learn about *zuo yuezi* until college, when my mom called to tell me that my aunt (her younger half-brother's wife) had given birth. My aunt's mother lived in Taiwan and was unable to travel, so she had paid a huge sum ($3000) to a local Chinese woman to move in and administer *zuo yuezi*. Of course, I was curious. My mother explained it to me, and I demanded to know why no one had done it for her. She told me that her mother had to work, so she didn't have anyone to help. As someone who always plans ahead, I asked her right then if, when I someday had a baby, she would do *zuo yuezi* for me if she could. My mother agreed, though she admitted that she had no idea how to do it.

A decade later, in a happy coincidence, my mother concluded her career as head of the math department at a high school in Southern California one month before my daughter was born. She contacted all her friends who had either administered *zuo yuezi* or had it administered to them. She began soaking the aforementioned black beans in rice wine.

I am thankful that I had the privilege of experiencing *zuo yuezi* three times with the support of my mother. I understand that others may not have that kind of help, so I included tips to encourage mothers trying to do *zuo yuezi* on their own or with limited assistance. Please don't get caught up in all the rules. The main principle is this: Take care of yourself, whatever that looks like.

I hope that any woman out there who is in need of help will seek it. Maria is involved with Postpartum Progress, a wonderful organization dedicated to raising awareness and support for women's postpartum mental health.

These Warrior Women are survivors who are fighting to change the perception that all women should be deliriously happy after childbirth, and that any other emotions are invalid. If you are hurting, please reach out. Let someone know. What you are feeling is normal. Do not be ashamed. Take care of yourself so you can take care of your child.

Lastly, I should be clear that doing *zuo yuezi* is by no means a panacea. Nothing is. But it worked for me, and I hope it works for you.

Guang Ming Whitley
April 22, 2016.

Chapter 1: The Basics

For over two thousand years, Chinese women have followed a tradition of postpartum recovery known as *zuo yuezi* or "sitting the month." The primary rule of *zuo yuezi* is confinement to the home for thirty days after giving birth. It involves a special diet, simple exercises, and a few lifestyle changes, all with the goal of encouraging the health of a new mother and baby. The Chinese culture is not the only one with specific postpartum practices meant to help a new mother, though they all seem to involve resting and soup.

In Korea, it is called *saam-chil-il*. It is three weeks of rest and seaweed soup three times a day. In Latin America, it is called *la cuarentena*. It involves 40 days of rest and vegetable soup. Unlike the cultural expectations in the United States, these longstanding practices recognize a mother's need for recovery after pregnancy and childbirth.

I experienced *zuo yuezi* three times: after the birth of my daughter in 2008, my son in 2010, and my identical twin boys in 2011. During each one, I ate foods meant to replenish nutrients leached from my body to support the growth of new life. I drank soups to promote the nutritional value and volume of my breast milk. I drank teas to flush toxins and excess fluids from my blood. I wore a special wrap around my torso to keep my organs in place while my doughy belly skin shrank back to (almost) normal. I did exercises from the comfort of my bed. I slept when my babies slept and ate every few hours. Following *zuo yuezi* was my only household responsibility. It was a special time of bonding, both for me and my children and for me and my mother.

By the end of each *zuo yuezi*, I had lost all but ten pounds of my pregnancy weight. I produced more than enough breast milk, even when the twins were at their most voracious. Most importantly, I never experienced so much as the baby blues. Each time *zuo yuezi* was over, I felt refreshed and energized – ready to take on the challenges of being a mother.

Not every woman has a supportive family or reasonable maternity leave. For these women, practicing *zuo yuezi* will seem daunting. Do not be discouraged. *Zuo yuezi*'s purpose is to encourage your postpartum recovery and should not be a source of stress. Find support where you can, and be willing to accept help. Be proud of whatever self-care you can accomplish on any given day, even something as simple as letting the dishes sit in the sink one more night so you can crawl into bed a little early.

Chapter 2: Lifestyle Commandments

1. Thou shall not leave the house.
2. Thou shall not have any visitors.
3. Thou shall not strain thy eyes with television, Internet, or books.
4. Thou shall not communicate via telephone.
5. Thou shall not be cold at any time.
6. Thou shall leave thy bed or couch only to care for thy infant or take care of thy bodily needs.
7. Thou shall not have sex.
8. Thou shall perform the exercises listed in Chapter 4.
9. Thou shall wear a cotton wrap around thy belly.

When my mother first informed me of the Lifestyle Commandments, I knew we were in for negotiations. I wouldn't have made it if all these rules had been fully enforced. It made me understand why many modern women consider *zuo yuezi* to be a burden, something to be endured to honor their heritage or the wishes of elderly relatives. At first glance, some of these restrictions seem arbitrary. As I worked to understand the justification for each commandment, I was able to offer alternatives that fulfilled the spirit, if not the letter, of the law.

<u>Thou shall not leave the house.</u>

The purpose of confinement is twofold:

1. To keep your newborn from being exposed to germs during his or her vulnerable first month of life, and
2. To encourage you to rest.

Infant mortality rates were high in ancient times, and this precaution saved lives in the absence of modern medicine. I asked that I be allowed to leave the house for doctor appointments, and my mother agreed.

My daughter had breathing issues at birth and spent her first seven days of life in the NICU. Because of this, my husband drove us to the hospital six times a day so I could nurse her. With the boys I only left the house to take them to their two day and two week appointments. All other errands were handled by my husband and (during *zuo yuezi* for the twins) my father.

If you don't have help, I would suggest limiting your trips out of the home to what is absolutely necessary. Rely on your spouse and friends to run errands. Order online if you can. If you have older children who need to be chauffeured, perhaps a classmate's parent could help with school pick up and drop off. Cancel lessons and schedule make-ups for after *zuo yuezi* is over.

While the thought of staying confined to your home that long may seem overwhelming, please remember the goal is for you to rest. It is only for thirty days.

<u>Thou shall not have any visitors.</u>

First of all, I need to define visitor. A visitor is someone who comes over to see and hold the baby and talk to you. A visitor gets comfortable on your couch. A visitor wants you to tell your birth story and asks how breastfeeding is going and how long the baby is sleeping at night. A visitor gives you unsolicited advice and expects you to listen attentively.

You spend time before a visitor comes making sure to cover up the bags under the bags under your eyes (there will be that many bags) and to change out of your pajamas. You miss all the cues your baby sends because you are too busy entertaining the visitor. When the visitor leaves, you will feel more exhausted than you thought possible.

Therefore, no visitors are allowed. I obeyed this commandment without argument and you should too. I knew that if I let even one person come over, the floodgates would open. Set clear boundaries while you are still pregnant. Enforce them. People with your best interests in mind will understand. Let them know that the minute your confinement is over, they are welcome to come over with a bottle of champagne and a hearty casserole. Until that time, you and your baby are off limits.

I was very fortunate to have all the help I needed with my mom. She cooked, cleaned, did laundry, and made sure I got naps every day. With the twins, my dad assisted wherever he was needed. He entertained my older children and changed more diapers than I did while singing his own version of Rocket Man (Diaper Man). I was lucky that my parents were retired when I started having children. Many women won't have the benefit of good helpers, especially not for an entire month.

Let's also be honest – even if you do have a

mother or mother-in-law staying for a while, she may not be that helpful. I have a friend whose mother refused to change diapers because she had "been there, done that." Another friend's mother-in-law spent her visit observing and criticizing: "Well, when John was a baby we [insert her way here] and he survived."

There are *zuo yuezi* specialists who will move in for the month. The price of this service has climbed from about $3000 when my aunt did *zuo yuezi* almost twenty years ago to over $10,000 plus food costs. Some women enter postpartum hotels, while others order a month's worth of prepared meals from *zuo yuezi* catering companies. These businesses are primarily Chinese language and only exist in cities with large Chinese populations. They are also very expensive.

So what do you do if you won't have a good helper staying with you for thirty days? Let the good helpers come over. A helper is someone who sends you and the baby to bed for a nap. The helper does your dishes, sweeps your floor and leaves a *zuo yuezi*-approved dish baking in the oven. She entertains your older kids and perhaps the baby while you sleep. After you wake up from your nap, the helper gives you a big hug and departs. The helper shows empathy, and knows that your sleep is continually interrupted overnight, your brain is hardly functioning, and your clothes are covered in spit up. The helper leaves you with fewer items on your to do list.

In order to get good helpers, you must be willing to ask for them. The person throwing your baby shower can provide little cards for people who want to give you the gift of help. Be sure to explain the *zuo yuezi* version of helping! If you make the "helpers welcome" part of your confinement clear, your friends will know there is a quid pro quo for getting to see the baby before everyone else.

Also, you don't need to exclude people who are coming to provide a necessary service. Since we moved to Alaska right before my son was born, I was home for the phone guy (twice), the cable guy, a security system guy (also twice), and a washer repairman. My mother had no objections.

If you still won't have help, only do what is necessary. Let dirty laundry pile up and only do a load when nobody has anything clean to wear. Folding it and putting it away? Ha. Let the floors and bathrooms get a little grimy. Make meals in batches so most of your cooking is just defrosting. Rely on your spouse to pick up the slack.

Thou shall not strain thy eyes with television, Internet, or books.

I am a woman of my generation. I love my

technology. I am also a total bookworm. When I was a child, my parents used to send me to my room for thirty minutes as punishment, and I would stay there reading for hours. Once they figured it out, my punishments would include a "no books" clause. So this commandment sounded just awful. A month of punishment.

My mother explained. She said that straining my eyes by doing any "close eye" activities during the first month would hurt my vision in the long run. I did some research and learned that the hormonal and metabolic changes during pregnancy can indeed change your eyesight, and it may take a few months postpartum for your vision to stabilize. So the eyestrain argument does make sense. Still, I asked for a few alternatives.

First, we have a big screen television so I informed her that watching it is not a "close eye" activity. My mother accepted this one rather quickly, in part because I don't think she wanted to go without television for a month either.

Second, I can't fall asleep at night unless I read for at least a little bit. She gave me ten minutes each night.

Third, if I couldn't surf the Internet, I wanted to at least be able to post some photos and updates for friends and family, especially since they had no other way of catching up with me. Again, she gave me ten minutes online each day via a desktop computer. No other form of online communication was allowed. She confiscated my phone because the screen was too small.

With my first two children, I used up my "close eye" time every day. With the twins, I was too tired. I discovered that I could indeed fall asleep without reading first.

If you have the willpower to follow this commandment completely, I applaud you. But don't be disappointed in yourself if you end up watching a lot of television. Once I had older children around, HGTV became the most entertaining of my daytime options. I watched whenever I was pumping milk for the twins. Apparently, I watched so much that my daughter, then age 3, informed me that our living room was too small, and we needed to push the wall back to open up the space.

Thou shall not communicate via telephone.

When you are engaged in a lengthy phone conversation, you are not paying attention to the needs of your baby, nor are you resting. My mother determined that I was allowed to take and make necessary calls, like setting doctor appointments and paying bills.

During my first two zuo *yuezi*, I was allowed ten

minutes per day of phone time with friends, though I did not always use it. For the twins, my mother changed the rule to zero phone time because she felt that I would be too tired to talk to anyone. She was right. Figuring out how to handle two babies at once plus two older children was a completely different and humbling experience.

<u>Thou shall not be cold at any time.</u>

Originally, this meant that the mother could not bathe for thirty days. Back then it made sense. There was no central heating or indoor plumbing. Being cold was associated with catching a cold. These days, only the most draconian of *zuo yuezi* administrators would forbid bathing. I just had to take hot showers and blow dry my hair right away. I washed my hands and brushed my teeth with water at room temperature. We kept the thermostat at 70 degrees.

When I left the house for doctor appointments, I dressed appropriate to the climate. Since my daughter was born in Los Angeles during the summer, I wore tank tops and shorts to the NICU. My boys were born in Alaska, with snow thick on the ground. For doctor appointments, I wore layers and bundled up in a down coat, hat, gloves, and scarf. I brought a thermos of hot tea to drink. My husband also dropped us off right at the entrance of the hospital so I would only be exposed to cold air for the ten-second walk into the building.

Thou shall leave thy bed or couch only to care for thy infant or take care of thy bodily needs.

Whether you give birth naturally or have a C-section, you will have some physical discomfort the first week or two. With my daughter, I needed a third degree episiotomy requiring an inch of stitches in a not so fun place. Lying down helped immensely with both the healing and the pain. Once she was released from the NICU, I camped out on our couch with a blanket and pillow. I only got up to eat, use the bathroom, nurse and change diapers.

Before my daughter, I struggled with the concept of *zuo yuezi* bed rest. I am strongly Type A, and I hate doing nothing. Then I had a baby. Then I had another baby. Then I had twins. Doing nothing is kind of nice.

My mother encouraged me to sleep as much as possible during the day. For the most part I had no trouble doing that. Even when I was unable to sleep, being on the couch forced me to rest. Otherwise, I would have been running around the house doing chores and crossing things off a to do list.

With my second and third *zuo yuezi*, my older

children learned to bring me books and toys if they wanted mommy playtime. If you won't have someone to help with your other children, you can buy yourself more rest by setting out snacks they can bring you for access. For example, stock individually packaged crackers, bars, and fruit leather or kid-sized plastic containers of cereal or dried fruit on a low shelf in your pantry. Keep string cheese and food pouches on the bottom shelf in the fridge.

About halfway through each *zuo yuezi* I got antsy. I felt better physically. I felt able to tackle my household duties. I felt guilty about the amount of work my mother was doing. My Type A nature threatened to rebel.

To keep me from going stir crazy, my mother indulged me with a single task per day, so long as it did not take more than an hour and was not physically challenging. I literally spent an afternoon organizing my recipe box. While watching HGTV.

Thou shall not have sex.

Whether you push a child out naturally (as I did with all four) or have it cut out of you, sex is the last thing on your mind after giving birth. In the ensuing weeks of sleep deprivation and adjustment to having a tiny, needy little bundle of joy, sex remains the last thing on your mind. Furthermore, most doctors do not allow sex until after the six-week postpartum checkup anyway. So this is a pretty easy rule to follow. If your husband is up for having sex during this time period, he is clearly not doing enough to help you.

Thou shall perform the exercises listed in Chapter 4.

After my first two pregnancies, I was able to do the *zuo yuezi* exercises as soon as my respective episiotomies healed. After the twins, I was not allowed to do stomach exercises because my muscles literally split down the middle of my abdomen (diastasis recti). This is fairly common with multiples and repeated pregnancies. The doctor warned me that I could give myself a hernia. So I waited for the medical all clear before attempting to regain my girlish figure. In conclusion, please consult your doctor before you begin the exercises set forth in Chapter 4.

Thou shall wear a cotton wrap around thy belly.

After giving birth, your skin does not magically snap back to its pre-pregnancy form. You still look about five months pregnant and your belly will be squishy like bread dough. My older children had tons of fun kneading my stomach after the twins were born.

During pregnancy, the growing baby displaces your organs. Once that space is no longer taken up, your organs pool at the bottom of your abdominal cavity. According to Chinese tradition, a cotton wrap keeps your organs from dropping permanently to new locations (causing a stomach pooch that will remain regardless of how much weight you lose or how many crunches you do).

You are supposed to wear the wrap for the first six weeks after birth – even beyond the confinement period. If you have had a C-section, wait until the wound has healed. I did not wear the wrap the first week after my daughter was born because my episiotomy hurt too much to get in the position needed to wrap properly. I was able to wear it right away after the boys.

In my experience, the wrap worked really well when my belly was soft mush. After about three weeks, my waist was no longer bigger than my hips and the wrap started to ride up around my rib cage. Since it no longer served a purpose, I stopped wearing it. You might need to wear it for a longer or shorter period of time depending on how your body responds.

While there are many post-pregnancy girdles on the market, they are all made out of materials with some stretch. Any stretch at all will allow your organs to pool. A better option is plain 100% cotton. You will need a strip 12 inches wide and 10 yards long. If you have a sewing machine, it is simple enough to buy a few yards of cloth and do it yourself.

If you don't sew, you can just buy 10 yards of fabric and cut it into strips. You would probably be able to make four wraps that way, though they will fray over time without hemming.

Put the wrap on after you shower in the morning and take it off after you brush your teeth at night to go to bed. If you are bemoaning a pooch from a previous pregnancy, know that each subsequent pregnancy resets the placement of your organs. The old pooch can be remedied!

Wrapping Instructions

1. Roll up the cloth like you would roll up a poster. Lying on your back, bring your knees up with your feet flat on the bed and close to your buttocks. Lift your pelvis and suck in your stomach. Begin with the wrap on top of your stomach.

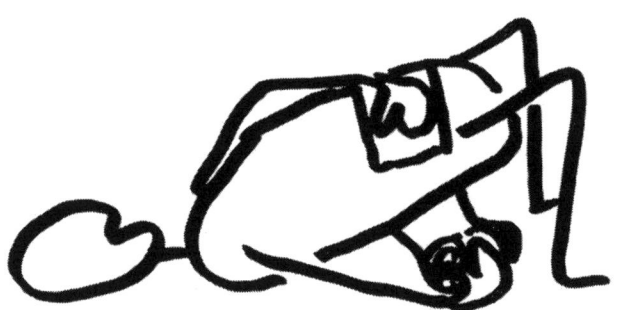

2. Wrap yourself (or have someone help) with the material, making sure it is nice and tight, but that you can breathe easily.

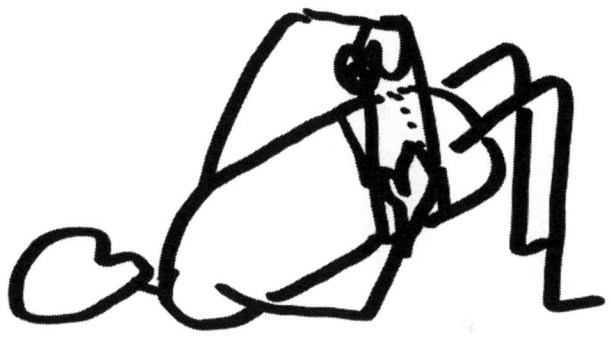

3. Every 1.5 times around your body, at the side of your waist, turn the roll of material over 180 degrees.

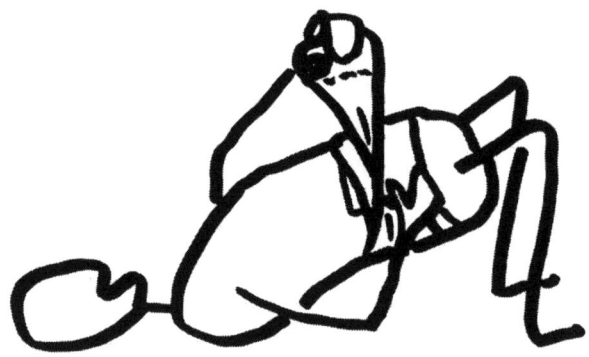

4. Continue to wrap. If you are doing it correctly, you will be flipping the roll on alternating sides of your body. The material should wind up and down your middle from the top of your hipbone to the base of your rib cage.

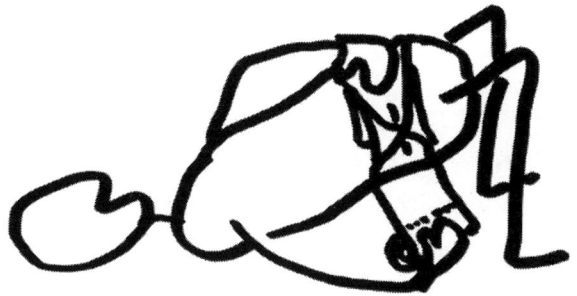

Chapter 3: Diet Commandments

1. Thou shall not consume salt.
2. Thou shall not consume chocolate.
3. Thou shall not consume any cold food or beverage.
4. Thou shall not consume caffeine.
5. Thou shall consume lots of liquids but not imbibe plain water.
6. Thou shall abide by the strictures of the food list in Chapter 5.

Thou shall not consume salt.

Because sodium causes water retention, eliminating salt from your diet helps your body flush all the extra fluids you have been carrying around throughout your pregnancy. Everything tastes bland at first, but soon, you will be able to taste the salt naturally present in meats, grains, and vegetables.

In following this rule, your diet will inherently be healthier. Severely reducing your salt intake basically means you cannot eat processed foods. Look at the sodium content of any canned soup or sauce and you will understand. You also cannot have any fast food or take out. To stem my cravings for the unhealthy stuff, I found it very satisfying to have a little something sweet at the end of every meal. Apple slices with almond butter. An oatmeal cookie. A sliver of pumpkin pie. As long as the treat is made without salt (and complies with the food list in Chapter 5) it is fine. Just don't go overboard or you will defeat the weight loss portion of the diet.

Thou shall not consume chocolate.

Chocolate is prohibited because it will cause gas in the immature digestive system of a breastfeeding newborn. This was a difficult rule for me to follow.

When not doing *zuo yuezi*, I keep a Costco-sized bag of Nestle chocolate chips in the freezer because frozen chocolate chips are delicious. I also used to keep a bowl of dark chocolates on the kitchen counter. After my older children became aware of its presence, I had to move it to the top cupboard. Sometimes they ask to smell my breath, just to be sure I'm not eating chocolate without them.

    Still, I managed to resist temptation. It was only for a month, and I had plenty of chocolate waiting for me when *zuo yuezi* was complete.

Thou shall not consume any cold food or beverage.

    This commandment goes hand in hand with the rule against being cold at any time. One of the goals of *zuo yuezi* is to flush all excess fluids and toxins from the body. According to Chinese tradition, consuming anything cold will slow down the process. This means no yogurt, soda, iced beverages, or frozen treats of any kind. Foods and beverages at room temperature are permitted. Foods and beverages that are hot are ideal.

Thou shall not consume caffeine.

If you are breastfeeding, the caffeine will go straight through you to your newborn, and a caffeinated baby makes mommy's life miserable. Caffeine can cause nervousness, shakiness, rapid heartbeat, insomnia and irritability. The cold rule already eliminates sodas and iced lattes (my favorite). The caffeine rule eliminates regular coffee and many teas. On the bright side, decaffeinated coffee is allowed in moderation. So at least I got to have the coffee flavor, if not the energy boost.

Thou shall consume lots of liquids but not imbibe plain water.

The historical rationale for this was lack of clean water supply. Teas and soups are made with water that has been boiled, which kills any lingering bacteria. While this rationale no longer applies today, I still followed this rule.

While doing *zuo yuezi*, I always had a large beverage container by my side and every meal included some kind of soup. I probably drank a gallon of herbal tea each day. My mom would make a large pitcher each morning, and it would be gone within 24 hours.

There are several types of tea that are part of

the *zuo yuezi* diet. They serve various purposes, including aiding digestion, replenishing nutrients, and flushing toxins from the body. If you are going to be drinking lots of liquids throughout the day (which also helps with breast milk production), they might as well be liquids with additional benefits.

Thou shall abide by the strictures of the food list in Chapter 5.

According to Chinese tradition, certain foods are "hot" while others are "cold." This has nothing to do with temperature, just the properties of a particular food. I have no idea if there is any medical evidence backing the designation of certain foods as cold or hot. I just obeyed, trusting a few thousand years of experimentation and noting that certain foods on the "cold" list are known to cause gas in babies (i.e. cabbage and melon).

Cold foods allegedly slow down the healing process, while hot foods are supposed to speed it up. Thus, during *zuo yuezi*, cold foods are not allowed. Chapter 5 contains a list with various consumables that are encouraged or forbidden. While the list is not exhaustive, the encouraged foods are diverse enough to keep your diet from getting monotonous.

Chapter 4: Exercises

These exercises are designed to help your body get back to where it was before pregnancy. Many of them can be done while lying in bed and are very easy to do. Be sure to do them on an empty stomach.

All of these exercises should be done slowly. Breathe deeply in through your nostrils and out through your mouth. Breathe in as you move from your base position. Breathe out as you return to your base position.

My mother drew the illustrations included here. Note that you do not have to be naked to do these exercises. Also, I took some liberties with the explanation sheet she wrote for me. English is my mother's second language; though I'm sure we all want to know how to "tighten vergina mustle."

Exercises in Bed (No Pillow)

Tummy Massage For Flush Duo
Begin on Day 1 of *zuo yuezi*:

    1. Lie on your back. Place your palms flat on your stomach, fingers pointing toward your toes. Slowly rub downward with firm pressure. Repeat 10x, 2x per day. This encourages flow of fluids and bowel movements.

    2. Lie on your back. Place your right palm flat on your stomach, fingers pointing to your left. Slowly rub your belly in a clockwise circular motion around your bellybutton with firm pressure. Repeat 10x, 2x per day. This also encourages flow of fluids and bowel movements.

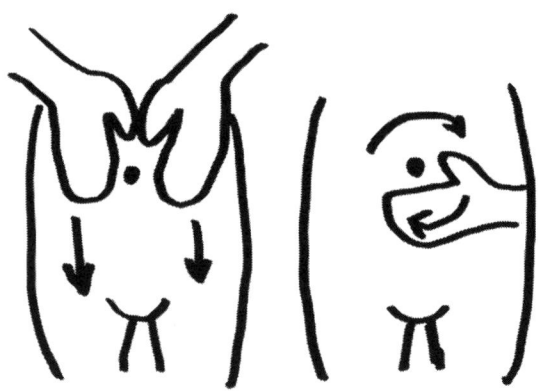

Deep Breathing For Tummy

Add on Day 2 of *zuo yuezi*: Lie on your back, keeping your legs straight and together. Place your arms at your side, palms down. Breathe in for 10 seconds, then hold for 2 seconds, then exhale for 10 seconds while trying to suck your bellybutton to your spine. Repeat 10x, 2x per day.

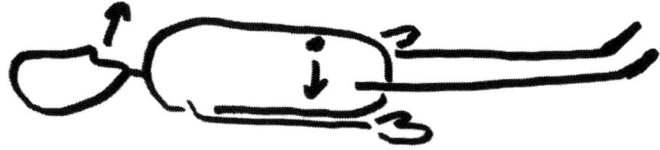

Improve No Saggy Breast

Add on Day 3 of *zuo yuezi*: Lie on your back, keeping your legs straight and together. Place your arms perpendicular to your body, palms facing upward. Keeping your arms straight, slowly raise them up until they meet at the center of your body. Clasp your palms together and hold for 1 second. Lower your arms to their original position. For the first week repeat 5x, 2x per day. Each week add an additional 5 repetitions until you reach 20x, 2x per day.

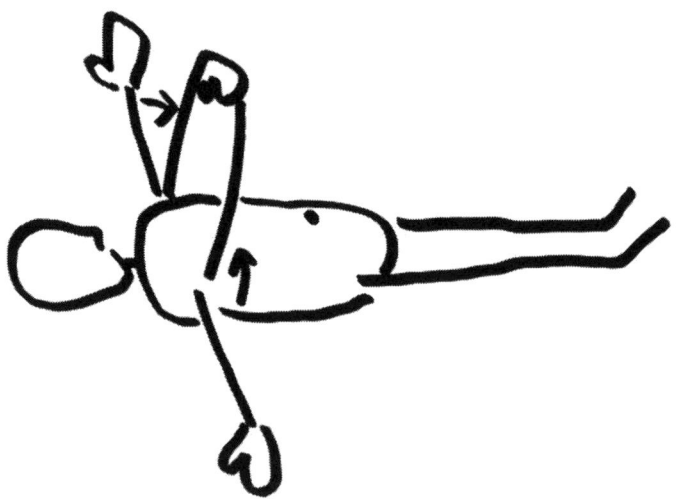

Slim Neck and Shoulders

Add on Day 4 of *zuo yuezi*: Lie on your back, keeping your legs straight and together. Raise your head, bring your chin to your chest on a count of three, then lower on a count of three. For the first week repeat 5x, 2x per day. Each week add an additional 5 repetitions until you reach 20x, 2x per day.

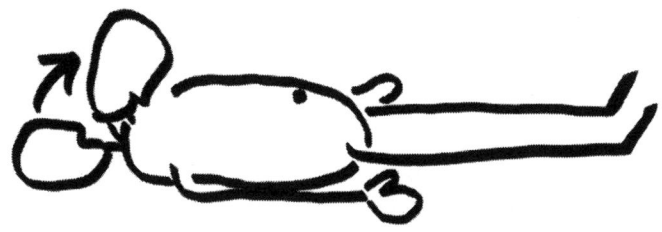

Flatten Tummy

Add on Day 5 of *zuo yuezi*: Lie on your back, keeping your legs straight and together. Lift one leg at a time to a 90-degree angle on a slow count of 5, and then lower on a count of 5. For the first week repeat 5x, 2x per day. Each week add an additional 5 repetitions until you reach 20x, 2x per day.

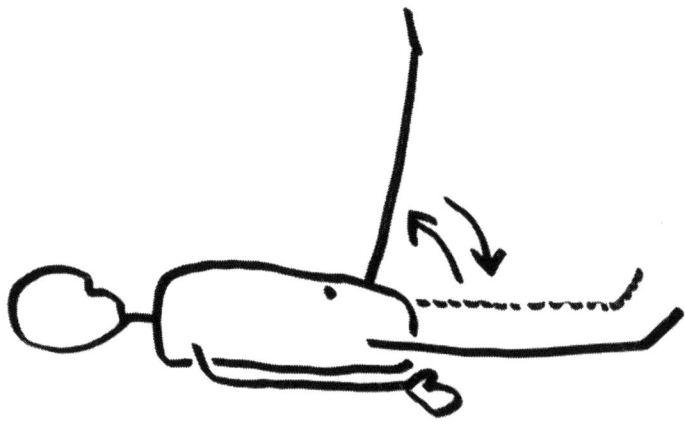

Get Rid of Big Fat Butt

Add on Day 8 of *zuo yuezi*: Lie on your back, keeping your legs straight and together. Bend one knee at a time, bringing it upward to your chest. Try to touch your heel to your butt, then return your leg to its original position. For the first week repeat 5x per leg, 2x per day. Each week add an additional 5 repetitions until you reach 20x, 2x per day.

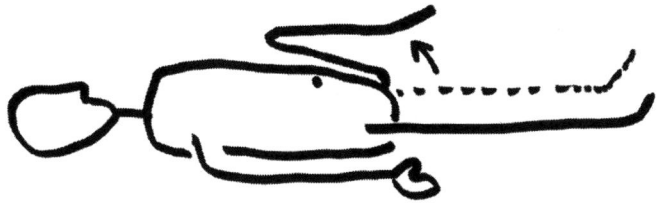

Tiny Waist

Add on Day 9 of *zuo yuezi*: Lie on your back with your arms perpendicular to your body, palms up. Bring your knees up and place your feet flat on the bed. While turning your head to the right, lean your knees to the left and hold for 1 second. Bring your knees and head back to center, then turn your head to the left and lean your knees to the right. For the first week repeat 5x, 2x per day. Each week add an additional 5 repetitions until you reach 20x, 2x per day.

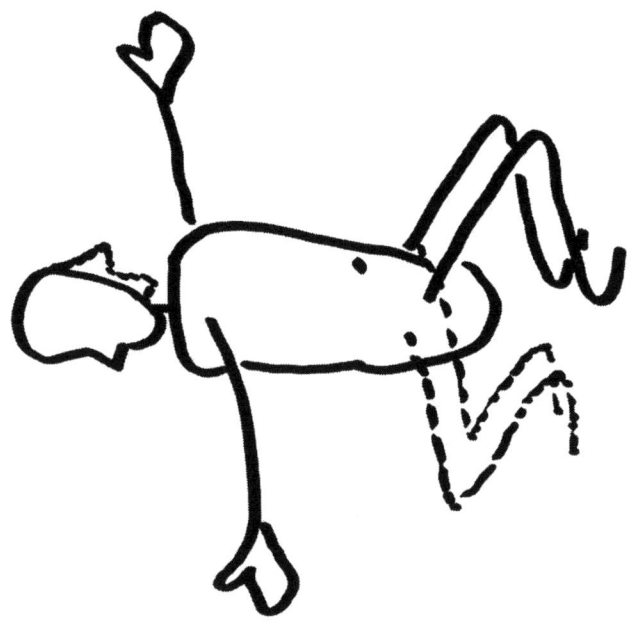

Tighten Vagina Muscle

Add after you have stopped bleeding: Lie on your back with your arms at your sides. Bring your knees up and place your feet flat on the bed. Raise your butt all the way off the bed on a five second count, then lower on a five second count. For the first week repeat 5x, 2x per day. Each week add an additional 5 repetitions until you reach 20x, 2x per day.

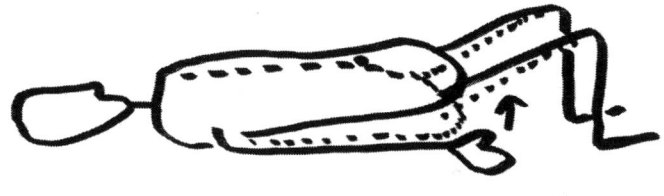

Exercises (Mostly) Sitting or Standing

The following exercises are a little more strenuous and should not be started until Day 15. Just add them to your routine. The entire process takes around 25 minutes and should be done twice per day if possible.

Slim Neck Trio (1)

Gently pat the right side of your neck 50 times with your left hand. Gently pat the left side of your neck 50 times with your right hand.

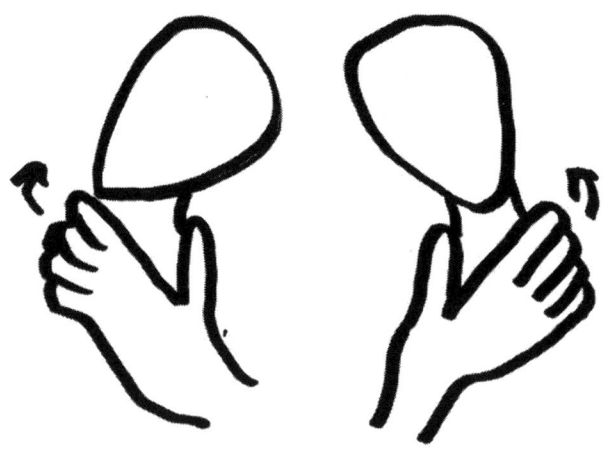

Slim Neck Trio (2)

Standing, hold your arms straight above your head, palms together. Tighten your bottom. Breathe slowly and deeply 3-5 times, then hold your breath while you lean backward. Hold this position and breathe slowly and deeply 3-5 times. Repeat 5 times.

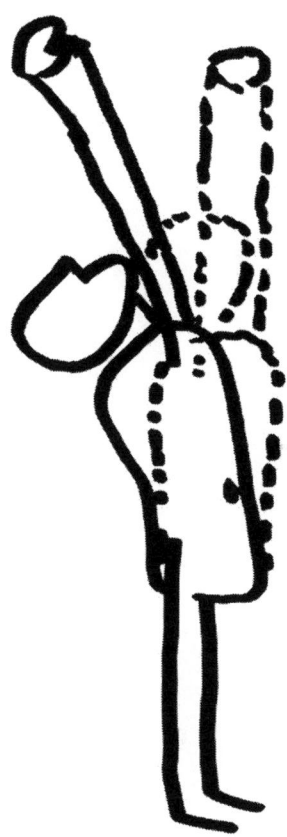

Slim Neck Trio (3)

Put your arms straight out, parallel to the ground so your body forms a T. Lift both palms as though you are pushing outward. Tilt your head to the right, back, and left, breathing slowly and deeply 3-5 times in each position. Repeat 5 times.

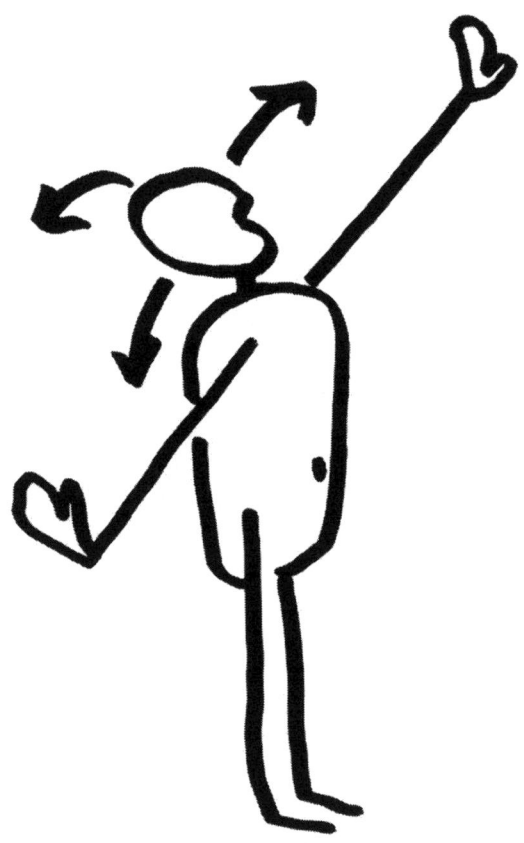

No Floppy Arm Skin Trio (1)

Sit with legs crossed. Pointing your elbow to the ceiling put your left palm flat on your back (if you can). Use your right hand to hold your left elbow, applying gentle pressure while pulling to the right. Breathe 3-5 times while holding this position. Switch arms. Repeat 5 times.

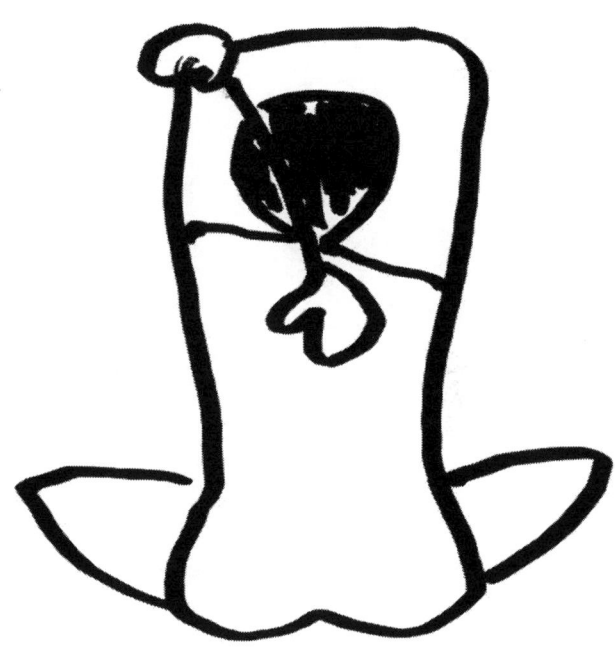

No Floppy Arm Skin Trio (2)

Sit with legs crossed. Raise your arms above your head and interlace your fingers, turning palms upwards to face the ceiling. Breathe 3-5 times holding the position. Bring your arms back down and rest your hands on your knees. Breathe 3-5 times holding the position. Repeat 10 times.

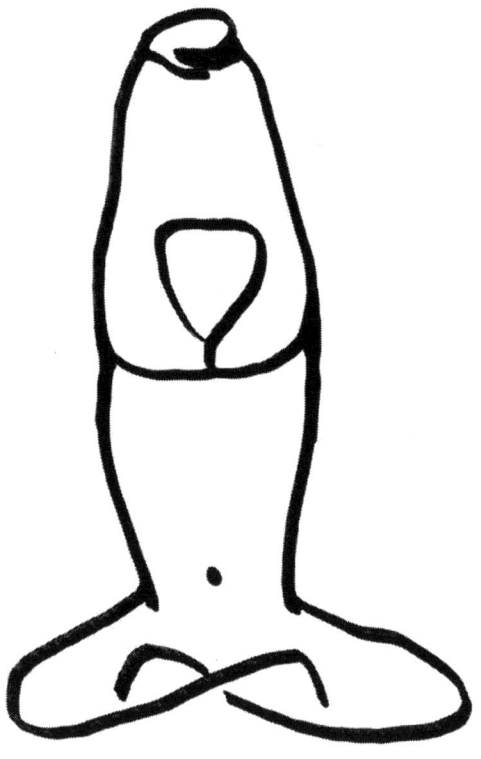

No Floppy Arm Skin Trio (3)

Kneel and rest your butt on your ankles. Put your left elbow in the crook of your right elbow and do your best to hold your palms together. (This was not physically possible for me. It looked really awkward.) Hold your breath and gently lean back. Breathe 3-5 times holding the position. Switch arms. Repeat 5 times.

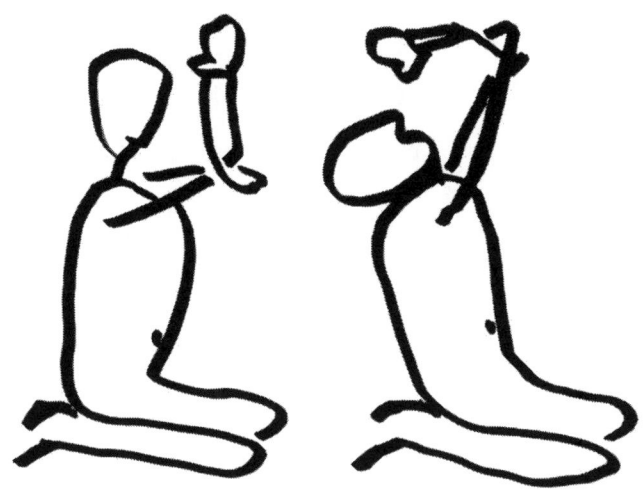

Skinny Waist Trio (1)

Standing up, clasp your hands above your head and turn your palms upwards to face the ceiling. Swing your hips to the left and right, breathing in and out with each move. Repeat 20 times. (I used to do this one while singing "Shake shake shake! Shake shake shake! Shake your booty! Shake your booty!")

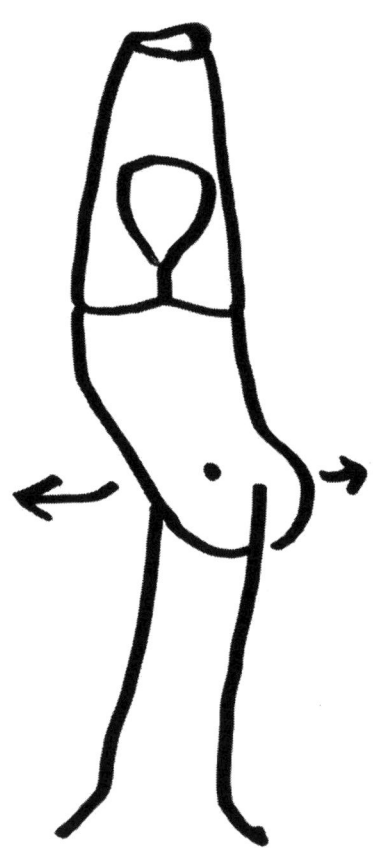

Skinny Waist Trio (2)

Standing up, clasp your hands above your head and turn your palms upwards to face the ceiling. Look up at your hands. Lean your upper body to the right. Breathe 3-5 times holding this position. Then repeat on the left side. Repeat 10 times.

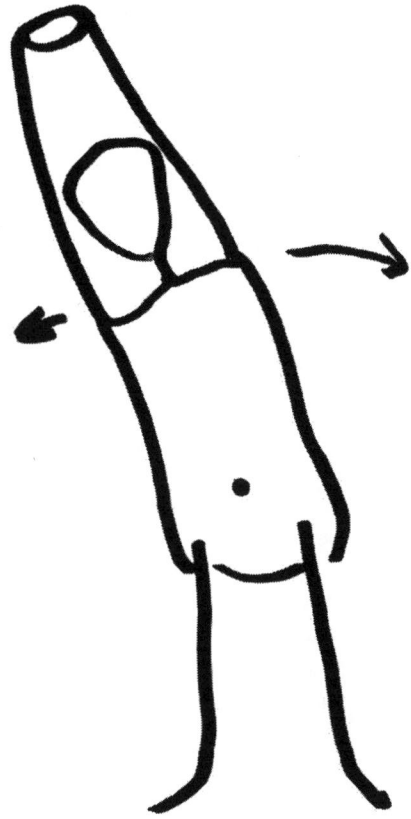

Skinny Waist Trio (3)

Stand with your feet slightly wider than shoulder width with both arms out to your sides, palms down. Bend over and touch your right foot with your left hand. Hold this position for five seconds while trying to look at the ceiling. Repeat on the other side. Repeat 10 times.

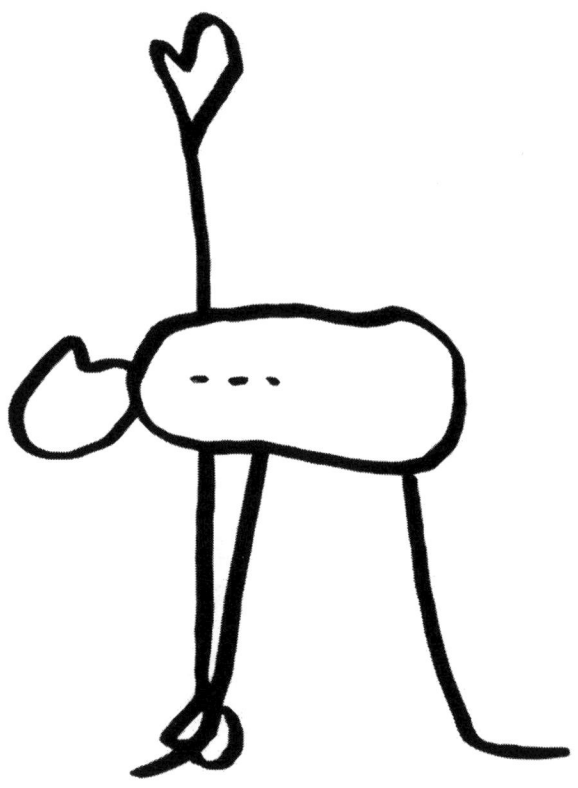

Flat Tummy Duo (1)

Kneel down with your hands on your waist. Use a yoga mat or perform the exercise on carpet to protect your knees. Breath in deeply. Holding your breath, lean your head back. Breath out leaning as far back as you can. Repeat 5 times.

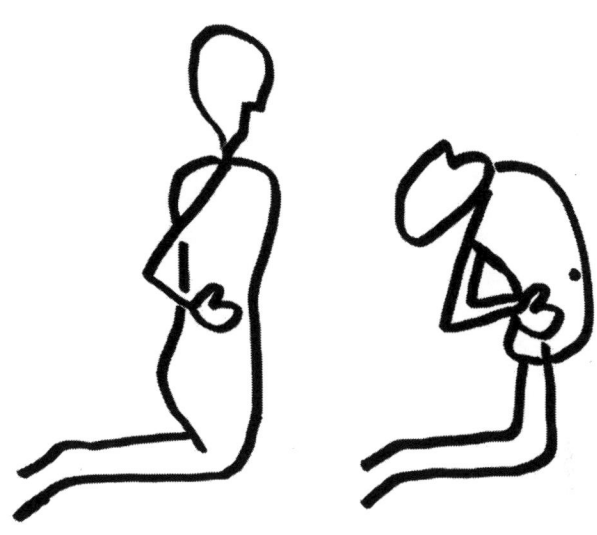

Flat Tummy Duo (2)

Lie on your stomach. Reach back and grab both ankles. Breathe in and tighten your butt as you raise your chest off the ground. Breathe 3-5 times while holding this position. Repeat 3 times.

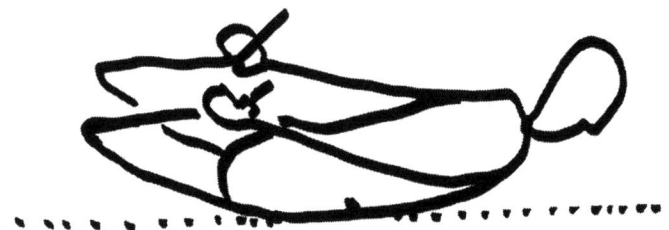

Improve No Saggy Breast Trio (1)

Kneel and rest your butt on your ankles. Put your palms together like you are praying. Pressing your palms together, keep your back straight and breathe 3-5 times. Repeat 10 times.

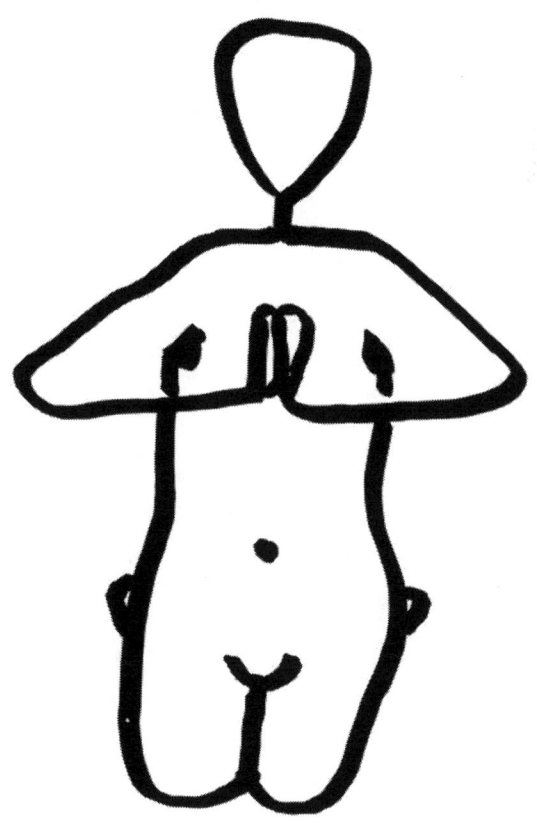

Improve No Saggy Breast Trio (2)

Kneel and rest your butt on your ankles. Reach back and rest your hands on your feet. Push your shoulders back and tilt your head back. Breathe 3-5 times holding this position. Repeat 10 times.

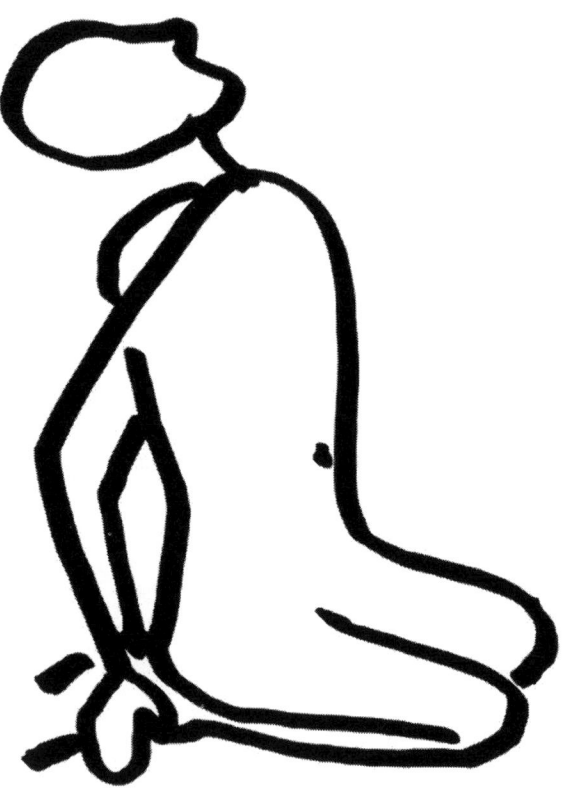

Improve No Saggy Breast Trio (3)

Sit with your legs crossed. Reach both hands behind your back and try to put your palms together like you are praying, fingers pointed toward the ceiling. (Again, this one was physically impossible for me to do. Just get as close as you can.) Breathe in and out 3-5 times. Repeat 5 times.

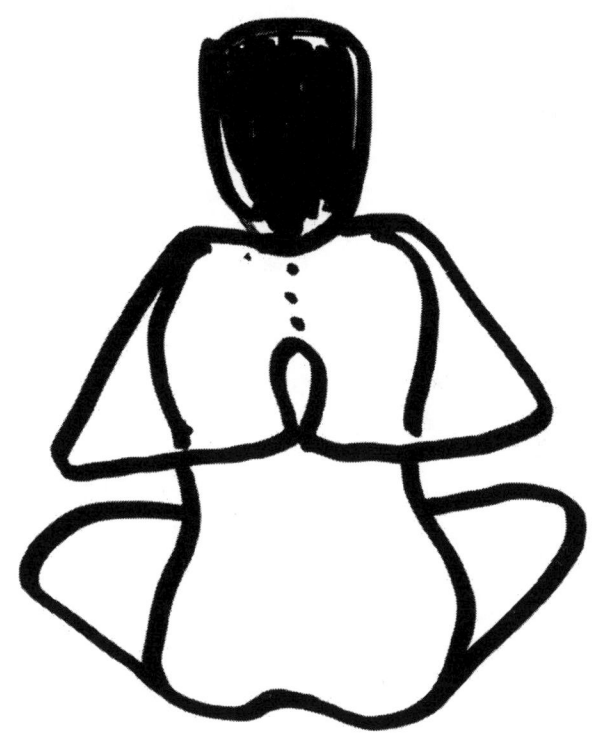

Shapely Calves Trio (1)

Standing up, put both hands on the back of a chair for support. Step back with your right leg and bend your left leg (knee should not pass your toes). Breathe 3-5 times while holding this position. Switch legs. Repeat 5 times for each leg.

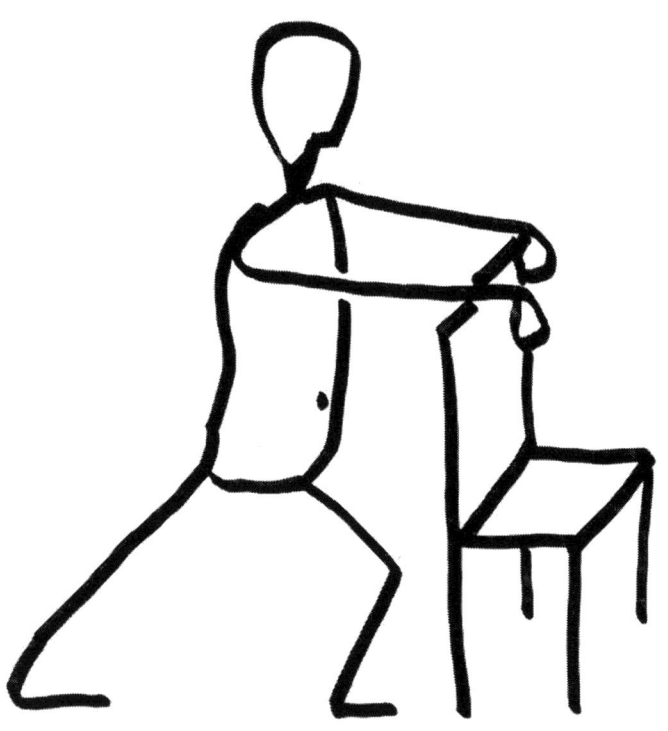

Shapely Calves Trio (2)

Sit in the butterfly position (bottoms of feet together). Holding your feet, lock your fingers together and lift your feet off the ground while straightening your knees as much as you can. Breathe 3-5 times in this position while sucking in your tummy. (This requires balance. I will admit I fell over more than once.) Repeat 5 times.

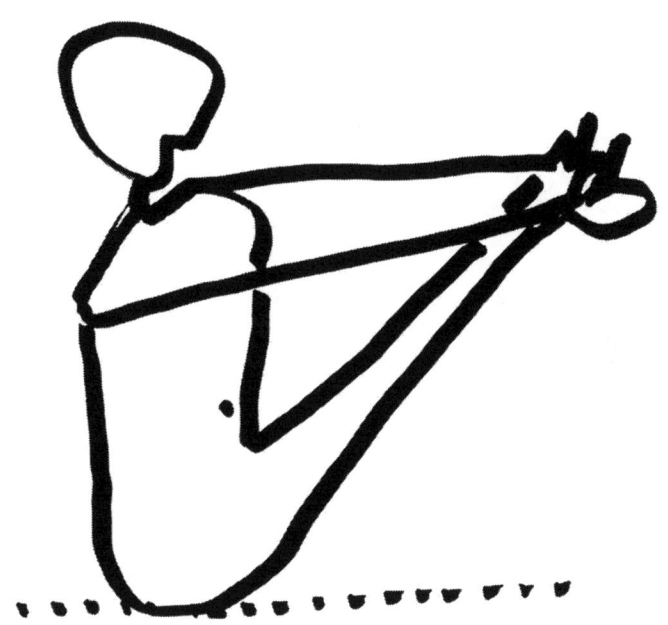

Shapely Calves Trio (3)

Sit with your legs straight out in front of you. Raise your arms above your head while breathing in. While breathing out, lean forward and reach past your toes with your hands. Breathe 3-5 times while holding this position. Repeat 10 times.

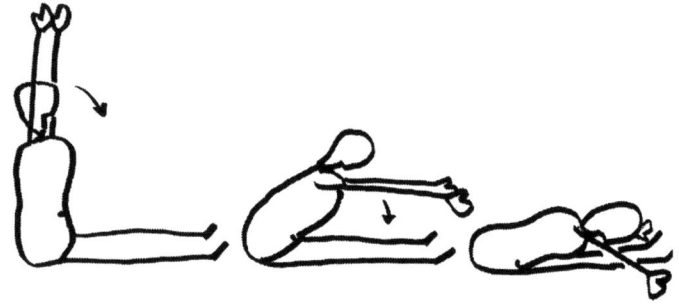

Get Rid of Big Fat Butt Trio (1)

Lie flat on your back and bring your knees up with your feet flat on the ground. Grab both ankles. Lift your pelvis off the ground. Breathe 3-5 times holding this position. Repeat 10 times.

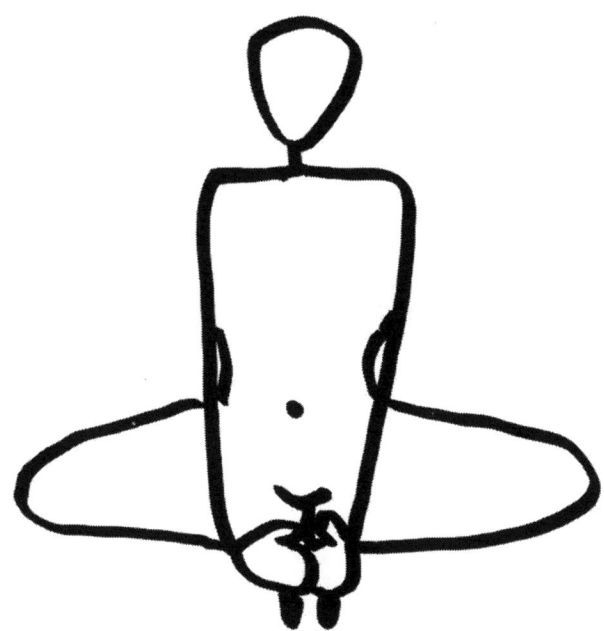

Get Rid of Big Fat Butt Trio (2)

Lie on your tummy with both hands stretched out above your head. Breath in. Raise both arms and feet off the ground as you breath out. Breathe 3-5 times holding this position. Repeat 5 times.

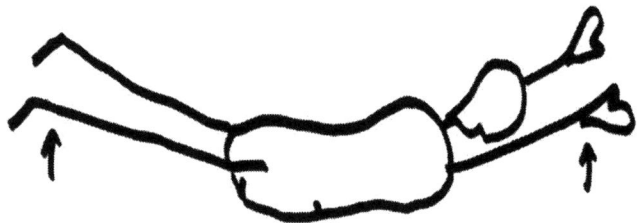

Get Rid of Big Fat Butt Trio (3)

Sit with legs crossed, right over left. Place your hands on the ground on either side of your body. Bend over and try to touch the floor with your head. Breathe 3-5 times holding this position. Switch which leg is on top and repeat. Repeat 5 times.

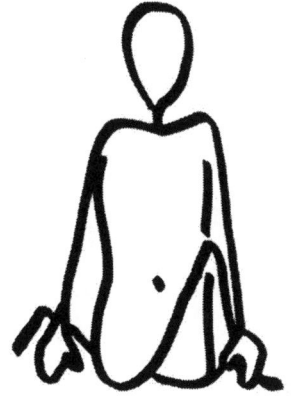 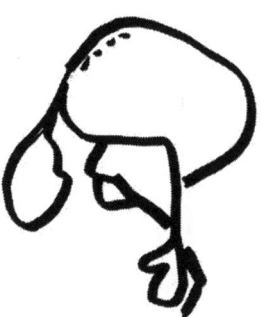

No Thunder Thighs Duo (1)

Stand up straight, both arms reaching straight above your head, palms together. Breathe in and slowly bend at the waist as far down as you can go while breathing out. Breathe 3-5 times while holding this position. Repeat 10 times.

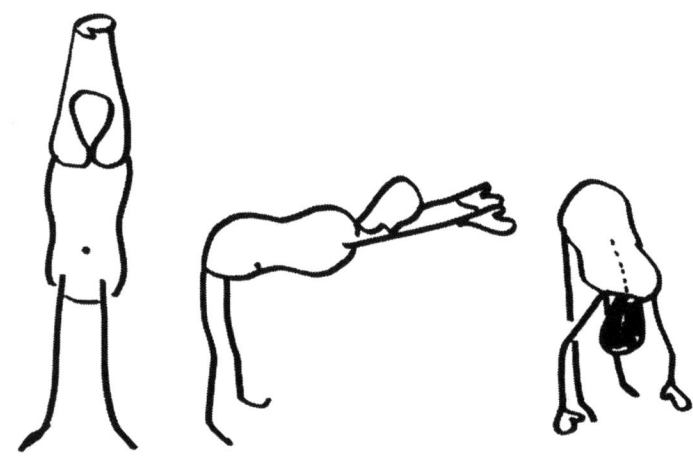

No Thunder Thighs Duo (2)

Stand up straight, both arms reaching straight above your head, palms together. Step back with your right foot. Breathe in. As you breathe out, bend at the waist to 90 degrees. Lift your right leg off the floor and look straight ahead. Breathe 3-5 times holding this position. Switch legs. Repeat 5 times. (This one also requires balance. Do not feel the need to do a beautiful arabesque. Just a little lift off the floor is fine.)

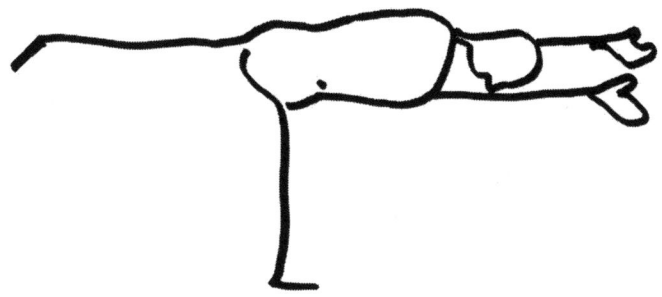

Chapter 5: Food List and Recipes

There are certain items that are essential to the success of *zuo yuezi*:

1. Rice cooker
2. Crock-pot
3. Electric kettle
4. Lots of single meal-sized storage containers with lids

Whether or not you will be making most of the food yourself, using the above items will make it so much easier. Having a large freezer is a bonus because you can begin stockpiling your *zuo yuezi* meals before you give birth. The electric kettle will give you a quick source of hot water for making tea. The rice and slow cookers can each hold 4-5 meal portions for a particular recipe. Because *zuo yuezi* involves eating six times a day, making multiple portions is a must.

Chinese mothers generally do not use recipes. Asking my mother how much ginger to add to her pork stir fry usually results in an exchange like this:

"Chop some up and put it in."

"How much?"

"Until it looks good."

So pinning her down on recipes for *zuo yuezi* was not easy. She got some "recipes" from her friends, but they were just a list of ingredients. Proportions and method of cooking were never explained other than a general understanding that frying happens in a wok and steaming happens in a rice cooker. I figured out the following recipes through a combination of observation and discussion. They are also only starting points for your own culinary creativity.

With the food list providing a guide to things you can and cannot eat, you can go wild with recipes. Substitute broccoli for spinach. Eliminate mushrooms because you hate them. Adding extra ginger "until it looks good" can really be whatever you want it to be.

While some of the ingredients in the recipes have specific health benefits according to Chinese tradition, the most important thing is that you are eating nutritious meals. So if you are not a fan of adzuki (red) bean soup (a breakfast porridge said to reduce swelling), eat oatmeal instead (promotes breast milk production). If you cringe at the thought of pig foot soup (the melted gelatin is supposed to regenerate your joints), use a bone-in pork chop. At least you will get the added iron from the marrow.

These kinds of substitutions are American Mother Alternatives (AMA), which I have included throughout the recipes. I just ate whatever my mother put in front of me, but then I have decades of experience with Chinese flavors and foods that are unfamiliar to the American palate.

Your local Asian market will have the various beans, grains, powders, rice and dried fruit found in the recipes below. Even Anchorage, Alaska has several small Asian markets, and while the prices are a bit higher than in Los Angeles, the items are at least available.

If your area has no Asian markets, try searching for the ingredients online or go with the AMA substitutions. How many Chinese recipes you incorporate into your daily meals is wholly up to you. It is possible to follow the diet without including a single Chinese recipe. To give you some ideas, I have included a sample menu after the food list.

During the first two weeks of *zuo yuezi*, you are strongly encouraged to eat offal: liver, kidney, and heart. Though the Chinese began this tradition before modern nutritional analysis, we now know that offal is incredibly high in vitamins and essential minerals.

Your growing baby took its sustenance from the food you ate and leached nutrients from your bones. Consuming offal gives you concentrated nutrient replacement. Depending on where you live, different kinds of offal will be available. Pork is best, followed by chicken and beef.

In my *zuo yuezi* experience, I had pork liver and kidneys with my daughter. With my sons I had beef and chicken livers because that was what was available in Alaska. I never ate heart and I did not miss the kidneys at all. I rather enjoyed the liver.

If the offal sounds, well, awful, you can rely on tofu, fish, and eggs for protein during the first weeks.

A final component of *zuo yuezi* involves Chinese herbs. Some of these are boiled for eight hours in a crock-pot until reduced to a terribly bitter concoction that is chugged from a shot glass three times a day for three days. Others are added to soups and teas. These herbs do not have English names. At least, they do not have English names that my mother was able to provide to me.

While these herbs are supposed to aid the healing process, *zuo yuezi* can be done successfully without them. When my son was born three weeks early, my mom flew from Los Angeles to Anchorage right away and did not have time to purchase all the herbs she used after the birth of my daughter. I did not notice a difference in my recovery, except that everything tasted better. Those herbs can be bitter.

If you really want to incorporate the herbs, I suggest that you visit your local Chinese herbalist, perhaps with the help of a Chinese-speaking friend. They most often work in Chinese supermarkets in areas with a large Chinese population. All you have to do is ask them for the *zuo yuezi* herbs and they should be able to give you what you need.

Hot (Good) Food List

Grains/Starches:
1. Adzuki (red) beans
2. Barley
3. Black beans
4. Kidney beans
5. Rice
6. Soybeans
7. Sweet potatoes
8. Yams
9. Wheat

Proteins:
1. Week 1: Liver and heart, pork foot, fish, tofu, eggs
2. Week 2: Add kidney, oxtail
3. Week 3-4: Add chicken, pork, beef, melted cheese, eel, shrimp

Vegetables
1. Broccoli
2. Carrots
3. Cauliflower
4. Celery
5. Corn
6. Mushrooms
7. Peas
8. Potatoes

9. Red bell peppers
10. Red onion
11. Taro root

Fruits/Nuts:
1. Almonds
2. Cashews
3. Lotus seeds
4. Raw peanuts (boiled until soft)
5. Cherries
6. Figs
7. Goji berries
8. Lychee
9. Longan
10. Loquats
11. Papaya
12. Peaches
13. Pumpkin
14. Red apples
15. Red grapes
16. Raisins

Beverages:
1. Coffee (decaf)
2. Black tea (decaf)
3. Chrysanthemum tea
4. Herbal teas
5. Red date tea
6. Goji berry tea

Cold (Bad) Food List

Grains/Starches:
1. Mung beans

Proteins:
2. Raw fish
3. Shellfish
4. Yogurt
5. Cold cheese

Vegetables:
1. Bean sprouts
2. Bamboo
3. Cabbage
4. Cucumber
5. Eggplant
6. Green beans
7. Green bell peppers
8. Tomato
9. Lettuce

Fruits/Nuts:
1. Banana
2. Green apples
3. Green grapes
4. Kiwi
5. Pear
6. Pineapple
7. Persimmon
8. Pomegranate

9. Any kind of melon
10. All citrus fruits

Beverages:
1. Caffeinated coffee
2. Caffeinated teas
3. Green tea

Sample Chinese Menu

Breakfast: 1 bowl longan egg soup
Snack 1: 1 bowl adzuki (red) bean purple/black sweet rice soup
Lunch: 1 bowl black bean and pork foot soup
Snack 2: Red apple slices with almond butter
Dinner: Pearl barley stir fry with liver
Snack 3: 1 bowl yam ginger soup
Beverage for the Day: Red date tea

Sample American Menu

Breakfast: 1 bowl oatmeal with dark brown sugar, cinnamon, and milk, 1 scrambled egg
Snack 1: 2 oatmeal cookies with raisins
Lunch: 1 bowl chicken noodle soup with carrots and celery (made with water, not stock, to eliminate salt)
Snack 2: 1 peach
Dinner: 1 grilled chicken breast seasoned with red onion, peas, and mashed potatoes
Snack 3: 1 slice warm pumpkin pie
Beverage for the Day: Decaf English breakfast tea

Recipes

Black Bean and Pork Foot Soup

Purpose: Good source of protein and gelatin, helps produce milk, strengthen bones, and repair blood

Ingredients:
8 ounces dried black beans, rinsed and sorted
1 pork foot (AMA = 1 bone in pork chop)
rice wine or sake (AMA = eliminate the rice wine/sake)
6 cups water

Directions:
Black Beans
The beans should be prepared 4-6 weeks in advance. You can also just soak the beans in water overnight, drain and add ½ cup rice wine to the soup.
1. Toast the dried beans in a pan on medium heat. Stir until hot and dry but not burned.
2. When cooled, place the beans in a glass jar or wine bottle and cover with rice wine. Put a lid on it.
3. Store in a dark place for 4-6 weeks.

Pork Foot

1. To prepare the pork foot, drop it into a pot of boiling water.
2. Stir to clean the foot for approximately 2 minutes, then discard the water.
3. Add the drained prepared beans (or unprepared beans and ½ cup rice wine) to the pot.
4. Add six cups water.
5. Heat on medium until boiling and then simmer for at least 1 hour. Can be done in a crock-pot.
6. Do not eat the foot, just the beans, soup, and any meat that comes off the foot.

Pork Foot Peanut Soup
Purpose: Increases breast milk production and assists joint recovery

Ingredients:
½ cup raw peanuts
1 pork foot (AMA = 1 bone in pork chop)
15 red dates (AMA = dried figs)
5 cups water
1 handful sliced dried shiitake mushrooms

1. Soak the peanuts in water overnight, then drain.
2. Soften the mushrooms in water at least one hour.
3. To prepare the pork foot, drop it into a pot of boiling water.
4. Stir to clean the foot for approximately 2 minutes, and then discard the water.
5. Put all ingredients in the rice cooker and turn it on.

Oxtail Soup

Purpose: Replenishes nutrients, helps flush toxins

Ingredients:
1 oxtail (AMA = beef short ribs, bone-in)
1 green papaya (AMA = cubed potatoes)
6 dried black dates (AMA = sliced carrots)
10 dried goji berries (AMA = peas)
2 cups rice wine (AMA = eliminate rice wine)
2 cups water
½ cup white lotus seeds (AMA = corn)

Directions:
1. Peel, seed, and cube papaya.
2. Boil and rinse oxtail bone in water for 2 minutes and drain.
3. Place all ingredients except goji berries in the crock-pot on high until boiling then reduce to low for 8 hours.
4. Add goji berries in the final hour of cooking.

Fish Soy Bean Soup
Purpose: Promotes nutritious breast milk

Ingredients:
½ cup soybeans (AMA = black or kidney beans)
¼ green papaya (AMA = cubed potatoes)
5 slices ginger
1 fish head (AMA = fish filet)
3 slices dried orange peel
½ cup rice wine (AMA = eliminate rice wine)
6 cups water

Directions:
1. Soak the soybeans in water overnight.
2. Peel, seed, and cube the papaya.
3. Shred the ginger.
4. Put all ingredients except fish and ginger into a pot.
5. Bring to a boil and simmer for 20 minutes.
6. Add fish and ginger and simmer for an additional 10 minutes.

Ginger Bass

Purpose: Repairs blood and helps heal stitches from episiotomy or C-section

Ingredients:
1 bass filet
5 slices fresh ginger
1 tablespoon sesame oil
rice wine

Directions:
1. Brown 5 slices ginger in sesame oil, then remove ginger.
2. Add bass and splash of rice wine and cook over medium heat until fish is white and flaky.
3. Add ginger back to the pot after the bass is finished cooking. Serve with rice.

Ginger Liver

Purpose: Helps flush uterine blood (should be eaten every day the first week after birth)

Ingredients:
8 ounces frozen liver
sweet potato powder or cornstarch
5 slices fresh ginger
1 tablespoon sesame oil
rice wine or sake

Directions:
1. Rinse the frozen liver in water
2. Thinly slice the liver while it is almost frozen.
3. Coat the liver in sweet potato powder or cornstarch.
4. Brown 5 slices fresh ginger in sesame oil.
5. Add liver and cook on high heat until done.
6. Add splash of rice wine and stir until evaporated.
7. Serve with rice.

Pearl Barley Stir Fry

Purpose: Lose water weight, flushes and strengthens your digestive system

Ingredients:
1 cup pearl barley
1 handful sliced dried shiitake mushrooms
½ cup peas
½ cup red bell pepper slices
1 tablespoon sesame oil

1. Wash and soak the pearl barley in water overnight.
2. Soften the mushrooms in water for at least 1 hour.
3. Dice softened mushrooms.
4. Cook barley in rice cooker with water filled to the 1 line marker.
5. Heat sesame oil in wok or pan.
6. Stir fry bell pepper, mushrooms, and peas for 3 minutes.
7. Add cooked barley and stir until mixed and heated through.

Variation for extra protein: Cook slices of liver or other meat in sesame oil first, then remove. Cook remaining ingredients as instructed and then add meat back in.

Time Saver: Cook the entire package of barley, filling the rice cooker to the appropriate number, i.e. with 3 cups barley fill to the 3 line marker. Save the leftover barley for later use.

Adzuki (Red) Bean and Purple/Black Sweet Rice Soup

Purpose: Reduces swelling softens and regulates bowel movements

Ingredients:
1 cup adzuki (red) beans (AMA = white rice, brown rice, or oatmeal)
1 cup purple/black sweet rice (AMA = white rice, brown rice, or oatmeal)
5 slices fresh ginger (AMA = cinnamon stick)
dark brown sugar

Directions:
1. Wash beans and rice, then soak in the crock-pot with 3 cups of water overnight.
2. Cook in the crock-pot on low for 6-8 hours and high for 4-6 hours until beans are soft.
3. After the beans are soft, add 5 slices fresh ginger and dark brown sugar to taste.

Adzuki (Red) Bean Rice Dumpling Soup

Purpose: Reduces swelling

Ingredients:
½ cup cooked adzuki (red) beans
1 cup water
20 rice dumplings
3 slices fresh ginger
dark brown sugar

Directions:
Rice Dumplings
1. Put 1 lb sweet rice flour into a bowl.
2. Add 1 cup water and stir until incorporated.
3. Adding water 1 tablespoon at a time, continue stirring until you reach a play dough consistency.
4. Pull off a chunk of dough and roll into a "worm" in your hand, approximately ¾ inch in diameter. Pinching off ¾ inch of dough at a time, roll into a ball and put on a cookie sheet.
5. After making all the dumplings, put the cookie sheet into the freezer for 30 minutes. Put the frozen dumplings into a freezer bag and use as needed.

Adzuki (Red) Beans
1. To prepare the beans, soak 1 lb adzuki (red) beans in water overnight.
2. Put soaked beans in crock-pot and cover with water.
3. Cook on low 6-8 hours or on high 4-6 hours until beans are soft.
4. Cool beans and store in plastic containers until needed.
5. The liquid from the beans should be saved and served hot in a mug with dark brown sugar and slices of ginger.

Soup
1. Boil 1 cup water.
2. Drop desired number of frozen dumplings into the water and continues to boil until the dumplings float to the top.
3. Add adzuki (red) beans and ginger and simmer for 5 minutes.
4. Add dark brown sugar to taste.

Yam Ginger Soup

Purpose: Helps immune system, provides fiber to prevent constipation

Ingredients:
2 cups yam, sliced into chunks
3 slices raw ginger, smashed
2 tablespoons rice wine
3-½ cups water

Directions:
1. Put all ingredients in a pot and bring to a boil.
2. Boil until yams are soft.
3. Add dark brown sugar to taste.
4. Yams may also be steamed, boiled, or baked first, which makes them easier to peel and cube.

Longan Egg Soup
Purpose: Repairs blood, gives strength

Ingredients:
1 ½ cups water
12 dried longan (AMA = 5 dried figs, quartered)
1-2 eggs

Directions:
1. Bring water to a boil over medium heat.
2. Add dried longan and boil for 2 minutes.
3. Add 1 or 2 eggs and gently stir.
4. Boil an additional 2-3 minutes until eggs are done.

White Sweet Rice Soup

Purpose: Provides strength, regulates bowel movements

Ingredients:
1 cup white sweet rice
1 cup adzuki (red) beans
1 cup raw peanuts (not roasted)

Directions:
1. Soak rice, beans, and peanuts in 4 ½ cups water overnight.
2. Cook in crock-pot on low for 6-8 hours or high for 4-6 hours until soft.
3. Add dark brown sugar to taste.

Mashed Taro Root
Purpose: Supports immune system

Ingredients:
½ taro root, cubed
Dark brown sugar

Directions:
1. Steam taro root until soft.
2. Mash and add dark brown sugar to taste.

Taro Root Soup
Purpose: Supports immune system

Ingredients:
1-cup purple or black sweet rice (AMA = 1 cup white or brown rice)
½ taro root, cut into large chunks
Splash rice wine
Dark brown sugar

Directions:
1. Soak the black sweet rice in 1 ½ cups water for at least 4 hours or overnight.
2. Put rice with water and wine into the rice cooker.
3. Place taro root in steamer basket in rice cooker.
4. Cook rice and taro in the rice cooker. When finished, peel and cube taro root, mix with the rice and add dark brown sugar to taste.
5. Taro root may also be boiled for 15-20 minutes until fork tender.

Barley Almond Powder Snack

Purpose: Lowers cholesterol, helps you lose water weight, helps regulate blood sugar

Ingredients:
½ teaspoon almond powder
2 tablespoons barley malt powder
1 cup water
honey

Directions:
1. Stir barley and almond powder together in a small pot.
2. Add a small amount of cold water and mix until lumps are gone.
3. Add 1 cup water and stir.
4. Heat mixture over low heat until boiling.
5. Boil for 1 minute, let cool slightly and add honey to taste.

Red Date Tea

Purpose: Flushes your system of toxins, rich in vitamins

Ingredients:
7 red dates with seeds
rice wine
hot water

Directions:
1. Make seven vertical cuts in the skin of each date, basically scoring it to allow the wine to soak in.
2. Soak red dates at least overnight in enough rice wine to cover the dates. To make things easier, you could use a large mason jar and soak an entire package of red dates and use as needed.
3. In small pot, combine dates and 1 ½ cups water.
4. Simmer for 1 hour with the lid on.

Goji Berry Tea

Purpose: Flushes your system of toxins, helps immune system

Ingredients:
1 handful dried goji berries
3 sliced dried or fresh orange peel
½ cup rice wine
3 cups water

Directions:
1. Place all ingredients into pot.
2. Boil until alcohol has evaporated.
3. Depending on strength of tea, dilute to taste.

Chrysanthemum Tea

Purpose: Flushes your system of toxins, aids digestion, replenishes nutrients

Ingredients:
1 handful dried chrysanthemums
5 cups water

Directions:
1. Boil water.
2. Add chrysanthemums and steep for 30 minutes.
3. Depending on strength of tea, dilute to taste.
4. May be sweetened with honey.

Impossible Pumpkin Pie

Purpose: Provides a sweet treat filled with Vitamin A and fiber

Ingredients:
2 eggs
2 tablespoons butter, melted
1 can evaporated milk (13 oz)
1 can pumpkin (15 oz – if you buy the larger 29 oz can, use half or make a double recipe)
2 ½ teaspoons pumpkin pie spice
2 teaspoons vanilla
½ cup Bisquick
¾ cup sugar

Directions:
1. Preheat oven to 350 degrees.
2. Beat all ingredients in a blender until smooth, approximately 1-2 minutes.
3. Pour into 1 or 2 pie tins depending on the size of your pie tins.
4. Bake 50 to 55 minutes, until knife inserted in the center comes out clean.

Oatmeal Cookies

Purpose: Provides a sweet treat packed with fiber and antioxidants

Ingredients:
½ cup butter, softened

1/3 cup dark brown sugar

1/3 cup light brown sugar

½ teaspoon vanilla extract

1 egg

¾ cup flour

½ teaspoon baking soda

½ teaspoon cinnamon

1 ½ cup oats (instant or rolled)

½ cup raisins (optional)

½ cup chopped walnuts (optional)

Directions:
1. Preheat oven to 350 degrees.
2. Cream butter and sugar.
3. Add egg and vanilla and beat until smooth.
4. Mix dry ingredients in a separate bowl.
5. Add dry ingredients to mixer and beat until incorporated.
6. Fold in raisins and nuts with a spatula.
7. Scoop cookies out with a tablespoon or cookie scoop onto a cookie sheet.

8. Bake for 10-12 minutes until brown at the edges.
9. Remove from oven and transfer to a rack to cool after 5 minutes.

RECIPE INDEX

Black Bean and Pork Foot Soup.	78
Pork Foot and Peanut Soup	80
Oxtail Soup.	81
Fish Soy Bean Soup	82
Ginger Bass	83
Ginger Liver.	84
Pearl Barley Stir Fry	85
Adzuki (Red) Bean Purple/Black Sweet Rice Soup	87
Adzuki (Red) Bean Rice Dumpling Soup.	88
Yam Ginger Soup	90
Longan Egg Soup	91
White Sweet Rice Soup	92
Mashed Taro Root	93
Taro Root Soup.	94
Barley Almond Powder Snack	95
Red Date Tea.	96
Goji Berry Tea	97
Chrysanthemum Tea.	98
Impossible Pumpkin Pie	99
Oatmeal Cookies.	100

Made in the USA
Columbia, SC
21 April 2025